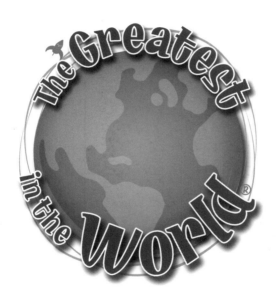

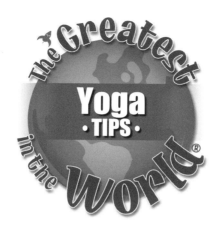

by

David Gellineau and David Robson

Illustrated by Graham Robson

Public Eye Publications

A Public Eye Publications Book

www.thegreatestintheworld.com

Illustrations:
Graham Robson, 'Drawing the Line'
info@dtline.co.uk

Cover design:
pentacorbig:
book & information graphic design
www.pentacorbig.co.uk

Layout design:
Bloomfield Ltd.

Copy editor:
Bronwyn Robertson
www.theartsva.com

Series creator / editor:
Steve Brookes

This first edition published in 20065 by
Public Eye Publications, PO Box 3182,
Stratford-upon-Avon, Warwickshire CV37 7XW

Text and Illustrations Copyright © 2006 - Public Eye Publications

'The Greatest in the World' Copyright © 2004 - Anne Brookes

A CIP catalogue record for this book is available from the British Library
ISBN 1-905151-07-1

Printed and bound by Biddles Books Limited, King's Lynn, Norfolk PE30 4LS

Acknowledgements

Through the practice of yoga I have been able to tap into unknown potential and hidden capabilities, both on and off the mat. This would not be possible without the guidance of my principal teacher, Ron Reid and my yoga buddy, David Robson, who has helped make this journey a wild, crazy and fun ride. I would also like to thank Marc Darby who inspired me to follow my dream.

I would like to especially thank Dad, Mom, Lisa and Spidey-aka-David, for their love, support and patience.

Sthira bhaga,

David G

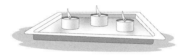

My students are my teachers, and my teachers are - well, they're my teachers too. My main teacher, Ron Reid, will always be my inspiration. I realise how lucky I am to be able to do what I love, and so I'd like to thank everyone who helps make that possible, especially my yoga-buddy, David G.

Most of all I would like to thank the beautiful, generous, and incredibly patient Miss Stan, who gives me unconditional love and support in any and every path that I tread.

Namaste,

David R

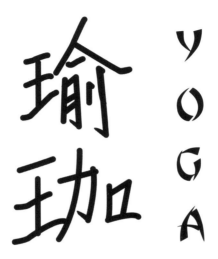

Contents

A few words from David G & David R . . .

Welcome to The Greatest Yoga Tips in the World. We have forged these tips on the anvils of our sweaty, muscled backs. Okay, maybe that is overstating it. Instead, let us say after thousands of hours of practice and teaching, we have gleaned the tips and facts that we are sure you will find useful in starting, or deepening, your yoga practice. The efficacy of these tips is guaranteed; we know they will work for you because they worked for us, either in our teaching, or our own practices.

When we first began to practise yoga, we would often do "yoga-thons", attending three or four classes a day. At first, it did not matter what type of yoga. We would attend any and all classes and workshops. We just loved to practise. Over time, and through experience, we became more discriminating. We came to understand what made a good class and how to distinguish a powerful teacher from an ineffectual one. We also learned what to do and what not to do when practising in a room full of other people, and a thousand other little details that can make all the difference in a yoga class. This book is our chance to pass on these discoveries to you.

Yoga has changed our lives for the better, and we believe that it can change your life too. We did not come to yoga with any pre-existing flexibility, great strength, or even particularly good health. Yoga has given us all of these things, and more. There is no yogic secret about how to obtain radiant health – you just have to practise. And practise, and practise.

We hope that you enjoy these tips.

Namaste.

David G   David RO

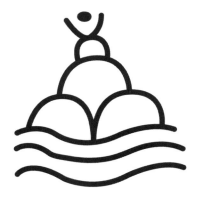

Health, Happiness and Peace of Mind

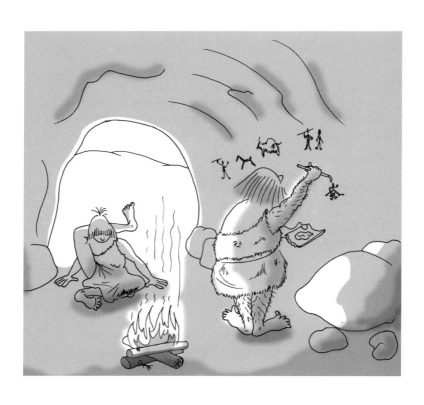

The Greatest Yoga Tips in the World

1. A Potted History of Yoga

1500 B.C.E. – The first archaeological evidence of Yoga's existence is found in stone seals excavated from the Indus valley, which depict figures sitting in yoga postures. These artifacts are from the great Indus-Sarasvati civilisation.

The *Vedas*, the sacred scriptures of Brahmanism and the basis of modern day Hinduism, also originate around this period. The *Vedas* contain the oldest recorded yogic teachings.

800 - 500 B.C.E. – The *Upanishads* appear. The *Upanishads* contained little that we would call yoga asana practice. Instead, yoga is described as a discipline or path to achieve liberation from suffering.

500 B.C.E. – The *Bhagavad-Gita*, a conversation between Prince Arjuna and Krishna, is the first scripture devoted entirely to yoga, and one of the most influential texts of Hinduism and yoga.

200 B.C.E. – Patanjali composed the *Yoga Sutras*, and defined Ashtanga, the classical eightfold yoga path.

9th - 10th century C.E. – Hatha yoga as we know it appears, as a development of Tantra.

14th century C.E. – The *Hatha Yoga Pradipika* appears, containing many of the postures and techniques that are used today.

1893 C.E. – Swami Vivekanada, a student of Ramakrishna, attended the Parliament of Religions in Chicago. He was extremely well received, and later toured the United States and Europe, proselytising the yoga tradition.

20th century - present – The 1960's and 1970's saw a renewed interest in yoga, and this interest has continued to grow. The practice of yoga, in a myriad of forms, thrives and continues to spread throughout the world today, with more people practising now than ever before.

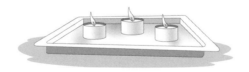

2. Yoga Traditions

There are many styles of Hatha Yoga, each with a different emphasis. No one style is necessarily better than another. Different people need different things from their practice. If you are thinking about taking up yoga, try as many different styles as possible. After three or four different classes, you will begin to get a clear idea of what you are looking for in a class.

Anusara Yoga
A new style of yoga founded by John Friend, Anusara Yoga combines heart-oriented philosophy with an asana practice that focuses on flow and alignment.

Ashtanga
Taught by Sri K. P. Jois of Mysore, India, this physically demanding style of yoga involves synchronizing the breath with a progressive series of postures — jumping from one posture to another to build heat, strength, flexibility and stamina. **Flow, Vinyasa** and **Power Yoga** are all variations on this method.

Hatha Yoga
Technically, all of these traditions are styles of Hatha Yoga. Recently, however, Hatha yoga has come to refer to a practice that is not necessarily associated to any one tradition. Hatha classes might include asanas, pranayama, philosophy and anything else that falls under the yoga umbrella.

Sivananda Yoga
Swami Sivananda set up ashrams and centers around the world that teach a traditional yoga system, combining asanas, pranayama, a vegetarian diet, positive thinking and meditation.

Jivamukti
Developed by David Life and Sharon Gannon, Jivamukti classes feature vinyasa-style asanas and also include chanting, meditation, music and philosophy.

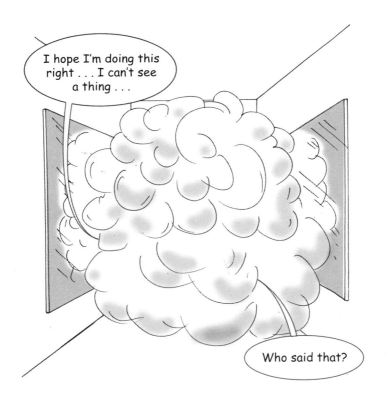

14

Bikram Yoga
A series of twenty-six asanas practised in front of mirrors, in a room with sauna-like heat. The heat makes one more flexible, and the sweat purifies the body.

Iyengar Yoga
Characterised by in-depth study of asanas and pranayama, Iyengar developed the use of props, like wooden blocks, chairs, blankets and belts that help the body into the asanas.

Kripalu Yoga
Developed by Amrit Desai, Kripalu Yoga encourages poses to arise spontaneously as practitioners work with their life force (prana) and create their own, unique practice.

Kundalini Yoga
Developed by Yogi Bhajan, Kundalini Yoga combines asana with breath work, chanting and meditation to awaken the mystical energy coiled at the base of the spine.

Partner Yoga
Two or more people work together to support and deepen yoga poses. Reliance on a partner develops and expands interpersonal boundaries and adds a new dimension to the traditionally inward work of yoga.

Viniyoga
Developed by T.K.V. Desikachar, son of the legendary Krishnamacharya. Viniyoga is an approach to yoga that adapts the various means and methods of practice to the unique needs of each individual.

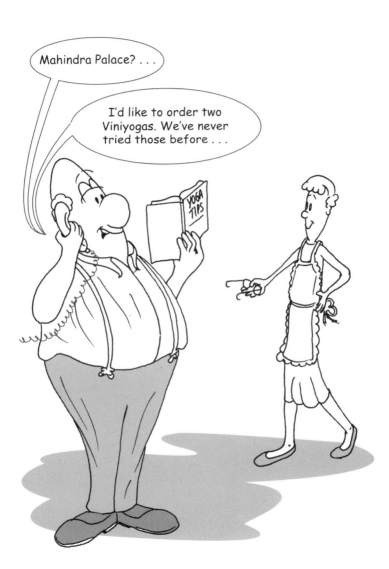

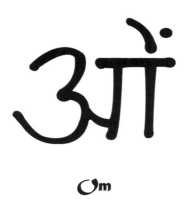

Om

3. A crash course in Yoga Philosophy

Ashtanga, the eight limbs
Yoga is more than just postures. In fact, postures are only one of the eight "limbs", or steps, that comprise the yogic path. The sage Patanjali first outlined the eight limbs in the Yoga Sutras, written around 2000 years ago.

While most of us are introduced to yoga through asanas, we soon realise that more than just physical changes come with our practice. The limbs of yoga guide us through these changes, directing our practice ever deeper and higher. The first four limbs deal with our external world, while the last four limbs focus on internal work and higher states of consciousness.

Yamas
The five Yamas, or "restraints", are ethical guidelines that address the yoga practitioner's behaviour, directing one to lead a simple and honest life. The Yamas are: **Ahimsa** (nonviolence), **Satya** (truthfulness), **Asteya** (nonstealing), **Brahmacharya** (sexual continence) and **Aparigraha** (noncovetousness).

Niyamas
While the Yamas address our behaviour towards others, Niyamas refer to behaviour towards one's own self, our spiritual discipline, or self-restraint. The five Niyamas are: **Saucha** (cleanliness), **Samtosa** (contentment), **Tapas** (heat, discipline in practice), **Svadhyaya** (study) and **Ishvara pranidhana** (surrender to God/the Universe).

Asana
Asana takes care of the body, our vehicle through this life. With the steady practice of Asana we gain the sensitivity and strength required to manifest the other seven limbs.

Pranayama

Pranayama is the practice of observing and ultimately controlling the breath. Early in our practice of yoga it becomes clear that the way we breathe reflects the state of our thoughts. By calming our breath, we can calm our mind and body. Pranayama is often practised with asana, but can also be practised on its own.

Pratyahara

Pratyahara is about consciously turning our focus inward, away from our external world. This is the practice of withdrawing our senses, not as an escape from the world, but as a step towards observing our inner self.

Dharana

Dharana is the practice of concentration. Maintaining pure concentration, even for a few seconds, can be very difficult. Yoga has many techniques to help us build our concentration, like focusing on a single object, repetitions of sounds and prayers, visualisation, and awareness of the breath, to name a few. Concentration builds as we use it, preparing us for meditation.

Dhyana

Meditation occurs when concentration is sustained for longer periods of time. When this happens, our thoughts become quiet, and our awareness is calm and even. Meditation is distinct from the process of concentration, in that we no longer focus on a single event in our field of awareness, but instead we become the field of awareness.

Samadhi

Samadhi is the final stage of yoga, enlightenment. Yoga aspires to reach this ultimate union.

4. Practice Tips

The Medical Bit

Consult your doctor before beginning yoga or any physical programme, to ensure that the exercises will not injure you.

Don't drink water

We have all heard about the benefits of a steady intake of water. It is true that water will keep our systems healthy, and most of us can definitely increase the amount that we drink through the day. That said, avoid drinking water during your yoga class, or at least minimise your intake. When we do yoga asanas, we build an internal heat that changes the body from within. Drinking water during class puts out the fire that you have been building, and diverts energy from your practice. Your body will have to devote energy to processing the water, instead of doing the asanas.

Water breaks are often just excuses for time out during class; you want to take a rest, so you reach for your bottle. Next time you need to rest, instead of drinking water try just slowing down your movements, so that you are only working at about 60% of your capacity. By focusing less on achieving the postures, and more on maintaining a calm breath and steady mind, you might find your thirst magically disappears.

If you still find yourself thirsty during the class, try to increase the amount of water you are drinking before and after.

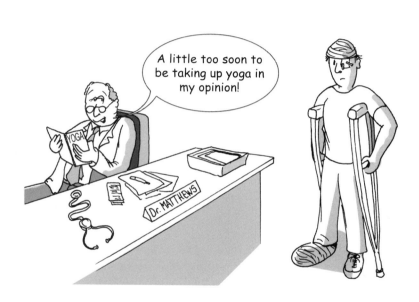

There is no winning

Yoga is not a sport. Your asana practice is your time to turn your attention inward, watching your breath, the sensations of the poses, and the movements of your mind. That is not to say that your practice will not contain struggle; no one does a calm handstand at first. But if you are trying to out-pretzel your neighbour, the chances are that you are not focused on your breath.

There is a saying that if yoga were about flexibility, then all gymnasts would be enlightened. Our outward poses do not actually reflect inward progress. We do asanas for a healthy body so that we can find peace of mind. When we try to impress others around us, we have lost the intention of our practice. So, instead of acting on competitive urges, try to witness them, recognise the urge to compete when it appears, and let it go. Turn your attention back to your breath, and remind yourself why it is you practise: to be happy and healthy.

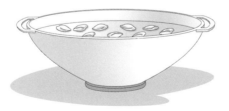

Monkey see, monkey do

When choosing a spot in class, set up beside someone who knows what they are doing. You will find that your practice will be easier beside someone who has a strong practice. Try to emulate whatever it is about their practice that seems good to you. This is a quick way to learn, as you can gain some of the benefits of their experience by simply aping them. It might be best to be discreet, though.

Another benefit of practising beside someone more experienced is that if, at some point, it is hard to understand or see your teacher, the chances are your neighbour might know what is going on.

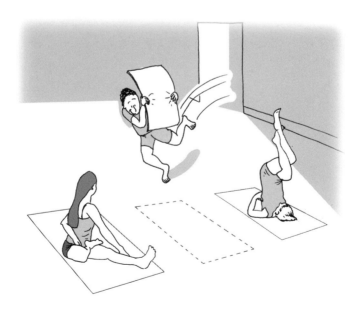

Settle on a teacher

Once you have decided on the style of yoga you are going to practise, you need to find a teacher. Or it might work the other way around - a special teacher brings you to a certain practice. Whichever way it goes for you, you should stay with one teacher as much as you can. Their teaching can be tailored to suit your specific needs.

Alternatively, beware of any teachers that demand too much of your time and/or money, who do not respect your limits, or make demands on you that you are not comfortable with. Let your teacher know how you feel right away if any adjustments cause you pain, or seem inappropriate.

When choosing teachers, try to get a feel for them. Do they embody the qualities that you seek to develop through your yoga practice? Do they practise what they preach?

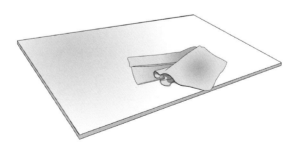

Choosing a teacher is not necessarily a lifelong commitment; it might not even be a yearlong commitment. Sometimes we outgrow our teachers, or our teachers go in new directions and we are not interested in following them. However, in the same way that you will gain the most benefit by committing to one style of yoga, you will learn quickest by studying with one teacher.

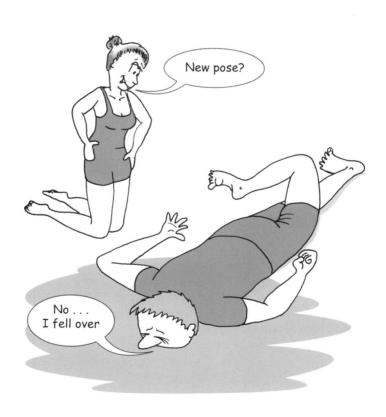

Control your hair

Long hair has to be kept up, or it gets in the way. If you are truly dedicated you should shave your head, but hair bands, headbands, and low ponytails seem to be more common solutions!

Keep a small towel handy

I keep a small, light, cotton towel by my mat when I practise. It is handy for wiping away sweat, and I also use it for grip on my legs in binding postures, which require me to wrap my arms around my legs. The towel can also take the place of a strap when you need a prop for forward bends - you wrap it around your feet and hold an edge in each hand.

Bring your practice off the mat

Yoga can give us the tools to be more present, and thus more mindful of our actions and their consequences. When you start doing yoga, you will almost immediately notice that aspects of your practice appear through the day, when you are off the mat. When you are confronted with difficulty through your day, use the same techniques that you would use when doing a difficult posture. Breathe deeply, try to relax and be aware of sensations in the body. Try to impartially witness thoughts and emotions. It is amazing how a few deep breaths can change your perspective on a situation.

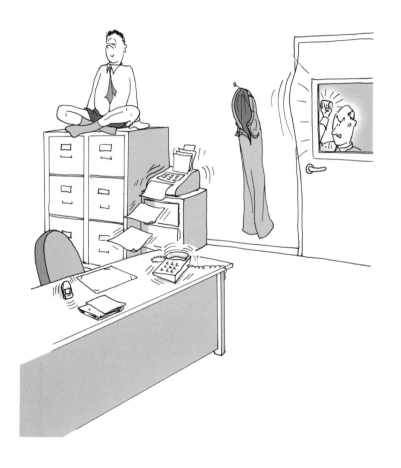

Lay off the moisturiser

Moisturiser and yoga do not mix. When you begin to perspire, moisturiser will make your skin extremely slippery. Not only does it become difficult to get a grip on your hands and feet, it also makes it very difficult for your teacher to give you adjustments. Wash any areas that you have moisturised with soap and water before you practise.

Cut your fingernails

Keep your fingernails trimmed, as you can give yourself nasty scratches.

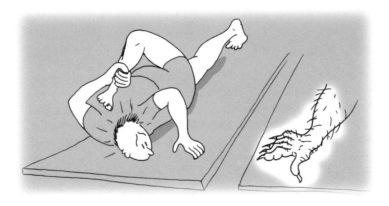

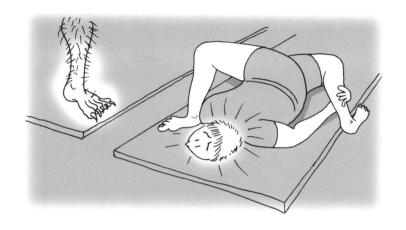

Get a pedicure

There are a few good reasons to take care of your feet when you do yoga. First, it is easy to scratch yourself if you have long toenails, and you can also gouge your mat. Second, when the dead skin on your feet accumulates, it will eventually crack. This can be quite painful, and so you should pumice your feet regularly. Finally, in yoga we spend a lot of time looking at our feet, and it can be quite demoralising to have to stare at toes that look like "dead pigeons", as one student characterised his feet.

The easiest solution: get a pedicure. It is not that expensive, all of the above foot issues will be addressed, and the treatment is quite relaxing

The Awakened State

5. Developing a Personal Practice at Home

Can't make it to the next yoga class?

We all have very busy lives and schedules, so finding the right yoga studio to attend and finding the time to go can be stressful. If you are unable to make it to the next yoga class, why not develop your own personal practice.

A great way to start the day

Choose the days that you will be practising. You might want to try Monday, Wednesday and Friday mornings. Most people think practising yoga in the afternoon or evening will be easier and will help them relax before bed. The most appropriate time for practising yoga is in the morning. This allows you to concentrate on your breath and move your body with effortlessness, as your mind is not cluttered by the day's events. The more yoga you practise the more energy you will have throughout the day.

Minimise distractions

Before you start to practise, get any immediate tasks out of the way, and turn off the phone, or promise yourself not to answer it. Commit to staying on your mat for the entire time you have set aside, even if you just sit there.

Create a space for your practice

To develop a self-practice, you need to create a space in your home and in your schedule. When you decide on a space in your home, roll out your mat in the same spot every time. Make sure that your practice space has enough room for you to move around without knocking into furniture. The space around you should be dust-free, and relatively quiet.

Once you have found a space in your home, you need to find space in your schedule. Be conservative with the time you need to practise; if you tell yourself you must practise for an hour, it will be hard for you to maintain the commitment. Start by setting aside 15 minutes a day. If you feel like doing more than 15 minutes once you are on the mat, gradually increase the time that you set aside. Be firm about maintaining that appointment with yourself. Once you have integrated your practice into your routine, it will be much easier to maintain.

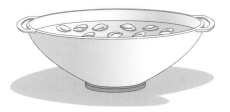

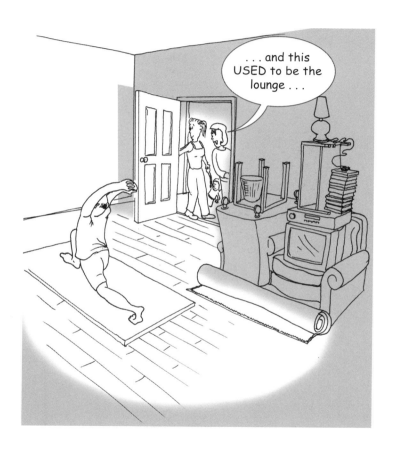

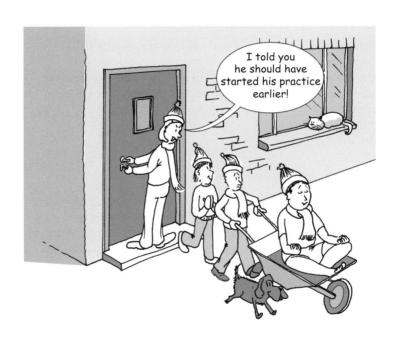

Stick to a practice routine

Left to our own devices, we will always focus on what comes easily, and avoid what is difficult and uncomfortable. If you come to yoga with a lot of upper body strength, you will favour arm balancing and avoid the poses that require opening the upper back and shoulders. If you have a flexible back, you will most likely shun the arm balances, and overdo the backbends.

Establish a balanced yoga routine that promotes work throughout the body. Unless you are already very knowledgeable about yoga poses, it is probably best to adopt a set routine from an existing tradition, or style, of your choice. Most systems have been designed by yoga masters, and will help you develop in a safe and even manner.

Build a ritual

Rituals are mindful routines, tasks that we use to heighten our awareness. Performing an easy ritual before your practice can help you adjust into a mood more conducive to yoga. Your ritual can be as simple as lighting a candle or some incense, or chanting an opening prayer, or even sweeping the floor around your mat. Whatever you choose to do, try to do it with conscious intention.

Check in with a teacher once in a while

As you progress with your home practice, try to check in
with a teacher at regular intervals. Correct alignment in the
poses is so important in maintaining a pain-free practice.
Often, we ourselves cannot tell that our alignment is off
in some of the poses. Imbalances in our bodies can lead
us to hold poses incorrectly, exacerbating the imbalances
themselves. A good teacher can see these imbalances in
your practice, and make suggestions for you to work on at
home.

Still the chatter in your mind

When self doubt and negative dialogue start to enter
your thoughts while exploring challenging postures, stay
focused on your breath and the sensations in the body.
Yoga stretches and asanas should be practised gently and
with correct breathing. Remember to practise compassion
and ahimsa (non-violence) towards yourself. If something
does not feel right then listen to your body's natural
intelligence. It is okay to talk to yourself, just as long as
you don't start answering.

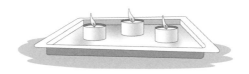

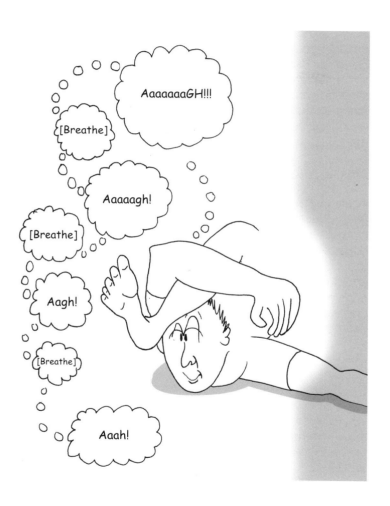

Feeling a little light-headed

If you are feeling dizzy or nauseous while practising, then stop!! The body has a way of letting us know when to stop practising and when to take a break and reapproach the practice. Part of getting stronger and practising is knowing when not to practise. If you can integrate this into your practice you will see quicker results. Remember your body has a natural intelligence that your mind can interfere with.

More isn't always better

Did you know that you can be too flexible? The major cause of injuries in Yoga practitioners is too much stretching. Too much stretching without strengthening might lead to injury. However if you combine both strengthening exercises and flexibility then you are on the right path to healthy flexibility.

Something to think about

Every action has a reaction. When you are practising your postures, stay present and active. Too often I have seen students become static in their practice. Try to find the deeper work in a posture that you are doing. You can do this by using resistance. For example if you are clasping your hands, try to pull your elbows to the sides. If your hand is on your chinbone, then press your hand against your chinbone. If you have become static or you do not feel anything in the posture, the chances are you are not practising with awareness.

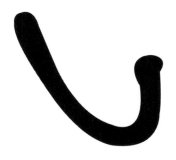

The State of Deep Sleep

6. Health and Diet Tips

It is true what they say - you are what you eat. Food is important for our bodies and it also has an effect on our minds. Sometimes we do not realise just how profoundly what we eat affects how we feel, until we start to eat properly and experience the transformation.

Vegetarianism

New yoga students always roll their eyes when I suggest going vegetarian. Really though, there are just so many good reasons to eliminate, or at least minimise, meat in your diet.

Countless studies have proved vegetarians often have a lower incidence of coronary artery disease, obesity, hypertension, and some forms of cancer. A balanced vegetarian diet will lead to balanced weight, making your asana practice that much easier.

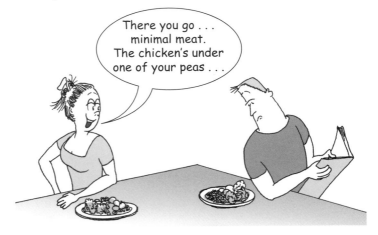

Balance your diet

If you are vegetarian, make sure that you replace the nutrients you were getting with meat. You can find plenty of protein in foods like nuts, whole grains, beans, and, if you are not a vegan, cheese. Also make sure you eat lots of fresh fruit and vegetables, either steamed or raw. Avoid processed foods as much as possible. Invest in your diet; spend the extra money for organic, fresh and natural foods.

Protein

Many people express worries about not getting enough protein with a meatless diet. A plant-based diet that includes a wide variety of whole foods will provide complete protein requirements. Western doctors report that protein deficiency is actually uncommon, and is seen mostly in countries where serious shortages of food exist and malnutrition is prevalent.

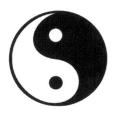

Ahimsa

From a yogic perspective, by choosing to go vegetarian you comply with the first Yama, Ahimsa, or nonviolence. You reduce the suffering and/or slaughter of animals. You also avoid accruing bad karma, which can pay off when the time comes for your next incarnation.

A yogic rule for eating is to fill half the stomach with food, one quarter with liquid, and leave the other quarter empty. Eating a little less than capacity keeps the mind sharp and the body light.

Allow three hours between eating and practice

Try not to eat anything for at least three hours before your asana practice. If you must eat, have something readily digestible such as fruit, yoghurt, or tea. It is also a good idea to wait for an hour after practice before eating.

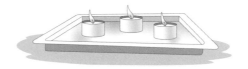

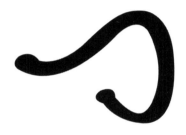

The State of Dream

7. Clothing Tips

Make sure your clothes fit

There is almost nothing worse than realising, five minutes into a class, that you are flashing your instructor and fellow students every time you lift your arms. Before class, put on your outfit and do some poses in front of the mirror. Stretch your arms into the air; do you feel comfortable about the skin that is exposed? Turn around and bend over; is anything hanging out? Sit on the floor and spread your legs; are you adequately covered?

It is important that you can relax and focus while you practise. If you worry about what you are wearing, you will not be able to enjoy the class.

Wear long pants for extra grip

Sometimes sweat can make it difficult to get your legs to stay on your arms in Crow Pose and Insect Pose. Long pants will help you keep your legs on your arms in arm balances, and will give you more grip when wrapping your arms around your legs in twisting poses.

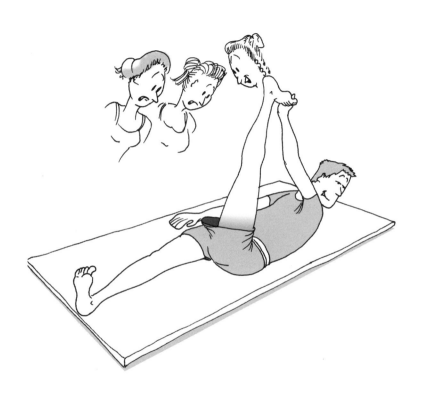

Avoid shirts that tie

There are many new styles of yoga tops available, but not all of them are good for all types of yoga. If you are practising a style of yoga that is vigorous, or causes you to sweat, then you ought to avoid shirts that tie up behind the neck. I myself have seen the shocking consequences of a poorly tied shirt. When the shirt gets wet from perspiration, the ties can come loose during vigorous poses like handstands. When you are doing an asana that requires you to balance on your hands, and then your shirt unties, unless you have a couple of extra arms like Siva, that shirt is coming off.

Bring a fleece or jacket

Bring something warm to put on for Savasana. If you have been sweating during your practice, you will feel a chill after lying still for a while. It will be much easier for you to relax completely when you are warm, and it is better for your muscles to cool gradually instead of quickly.

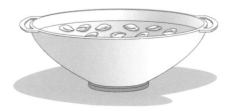

Tight clothes are better than loose ones

Loose clothes will get in your way during postures. Loose pants will bag around the thighs during inversions, and loose shirts will ride up to your chin. It will also be difficult for your teacher to see your alignment when you wear baggy clothes. It is much wiser to wear tight, stretchy clothes that fit close to your body.

Add vinegar to your yoga wash

Yoga outfits tend to be damp for long periods of time, and can develop mildewed odours that become difficult to get rid of with a regular wash. Ensure that your clothes dry before putting them in the laundry basket. Also, try putting two cups of vinegar in the rinse cycle of your wash and the mildew smell should disappear.

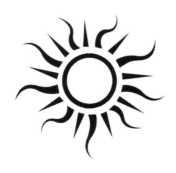

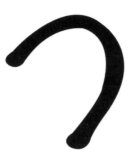

The Ordinary or Material State

8. Mat tips

The best mat

The mat you need will depend on the type of yoga, and how often you practise. As the popularity of yoga has increased, so have your options in mat purchases. Unfortunately, many of the mats now on sale are practically disposable, as they start to deteriorate very quickly.

If you're practising regularly, it is best to invest in a sturdy mat; a thick, dense mat is generally best. The thicker the mat, the less you will feel the floor under you, and this can be especially important for the knees and the spine. If the mat is too soft, it will not give your wrists enough support when you press into your hands. Soft mats also tend to start shredding quickly.

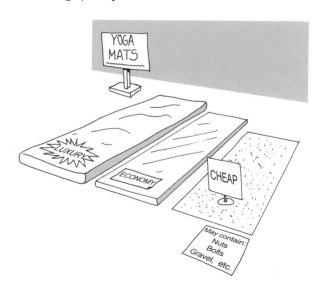

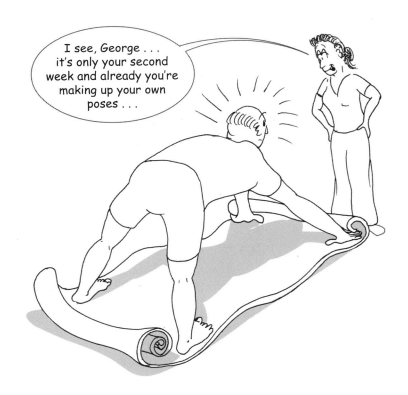

Align your mat

Make sure your mat is straight when you lay it down by aligning it to the floorboards or wall. Keeping yourself straight on your mat becomes easier when your mat is straight, too.

Stagger your mat for more room

When the class is crowded, place your mat a few inches in front or behind your neighbour's mat. This way, you will have room to raise your arms out to the sides, spread your legs, etc.

Stand off the mat for more balance

Sometimes the cushion of even a thin mat can make it difficult to balance on one leg. Try stepping off the mat and you will find it easier to balance.

Roll your mat opposite to the curl

If you roll your mat opposite to its existing curl, the next time you unroll your mat it will stay flat.

Use a rug for more traction

Some types of yoga can make you very sweaty, and rubber mats can become slippery. The best solution is to put down a thin cotton rug, specially sized to your yoga mat, which you can purchase either online or through some yoga studios. The rug works best once the mat is already a little damp. If you are not a producing enough sweat to keep the rug on your mat, spray a little water on the rug when you first lay it down.

Wash your mat for more grip, less stink

New mats are often coated with a thin plastic film that can make them very slippery. There can also be a very strong plastic smell. To get rid of both of these problems, just pop your mat in the wash. Most sticky mats can be put into the washing machine at a low temperature. This works when your mat gets stinky from use, too. Just make sure you hang your mat to dry and do not put it in a dryer.

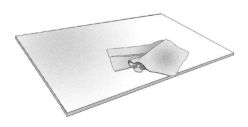

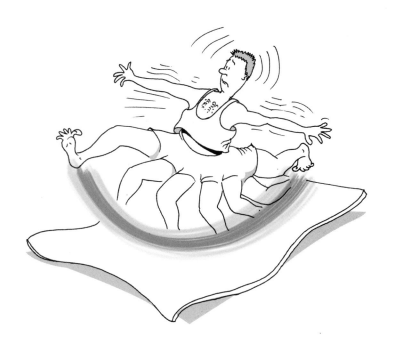

Clean your mat regularly

All mats will tend to pick up odours over time. How often you clean your mat is up to you. The more you sweat during your practice, the more often you should give your mat a scrub. Since your skin will be coming into contact with the mat, make sure to use a natural cleaning product, or make your own. Here is an easy recipe for a natural anti-bacterial cleanser:

- Fill an empty spray bottle almost to the top with equal parts vinegar and water
- Add 4 tbsp of lemon juice
- Add 1 tbsp of tea tree oil or lavender oil

Put a strap across the mat for more grip

Slippery mats and wet hands make a frustrating combination, especially in poses like Downward-Facing Dog. Some people bring hand towels to class, and put these across the front of their mats to provide some grip. If you have not brought a hand towel, use a yoga strap. Almost all yoga studios have their own supply of straps. Place a doubled strap across the front of your mat, with the straps running parallel and about an inch apart. The straps will provide extra grip for your hands without getting in the way, and there is no extra laundry when you get home.

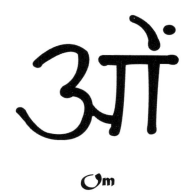

Om

9. Basic Alignment Principles

When we begin to practise yoga we begin to change or correct the damage that everyday life can put on our bodies. In essence we begin to physically evolve. With this in mind there are basic alignment principals and movements to remember when practising. By understanding how your body moves you can merge different movements together to perform a yoga posture. The following are basic movements of the body and the foundation for your yoga postures.

1. Abduction and Adduction
Abduction occurs when you move a limb away from the midline, while adduction moves the limb towards the midline, or returns from abduction.

2. Flexion and Extension
Flexion usually occurs when you bend a limb or joint, while extension returns the limb back after it has been bent.

3. Medial and Lateral Rotations
Medial and lateral rotations are also known as internal and external rotations. Medial (internal) rotations occur when you rotate towards your midline and lateral (external) rotations occur when you rotate away from your midline.

All the movements of the body are made up of components of these basic movements. There are other directions, actions and intricate combinations of movements of the body; however they become more individual depending on your body type. These movements may aid or limit us from moving into the full extension or a deeper version of a posture, e.g. hyperextension.

Hyperextension is the movement of a limb or joint beyond the normal range of motion. A person may hyperextend their forearm or chinbone. So their movements will be different from someone who doesn't hyperextend. You will discover when you start to practise that some postures are easier, while some are more challenging. The reason for this can usually be found in one of the six basic movements of the body.

Keep in mind when practising yoga postures you are trying to correct or realign your body. If something is challenging at first, practise intelligently and consistently until your body has assimilated the information and eventually realigns itself. Never force yourself to the point of pain or injury. A good way to measure if you are approaching a place of discomfort is your breath. If you are finding it difficult to breath then pull back, regain control of your breath and re-approach your practice. One of the goals of yoga postures is to restore the body to its natural state and enhance your life.

10. The Practice

The next section outlines a suggested sequence and tips for the more familiar, classic Hatha yoga postures. Before you begin, read each posture and tip to familiarise yourself with the instructions. I have also included the Sanskrit to English translation. Learn the name of each posture. A wise Yogi once said to me "If you don't know the name of the postures then you cannot understand or do them".

This section also outlines some of the therapeutic benefits that have been shown to arise from regularly practising the postures. Before we begin I would like to say that therapeutic benefits take time to work and do not replace the advice given to you by a medical doctor. Always consult your family doctor.

Remember to hold each posture for five breaths and then release. As your practice deepens you will be able to hold the postures for longer periods.

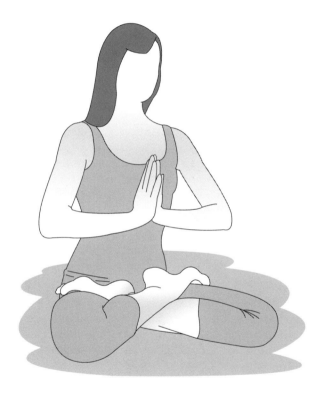

Lotus

The Classic Asanas

Standing Postures

Standing postures help strengthen the legs and the pelvic region. They are also the foundation of every yoga posture. All yoga postures start with the feet and move up the entire body to the crown of the head.

Tadasana (Mountain Posture)

"Tada" means mountain.

1. Bend your knees and come into a squatting position, then, pressing the feet into the floor, slowly straighten your legs; this will help you find the actions of your legs and ensure that you are standing evenly on both legs.

2. Bring your anklebones together. This will help to rotate the thighs in.

3. Lift and spread your toes. Now lower them onto the mat.

4. Lean the weight forward into the toes. Now lean the weight back into your heels. This will help ensure that you are standing on all eight corners of your feet.

5. Keep the head upright and find a spot to gaze at. Pick a spot on the floor, approximately three feet in front of you, to help you focus. Tuck your chin slightly to help lengthen the back of the neck. Lift the navel and keep your pelvis in neutral.

6. Let the shoulders drop away from the ears and the arms rest by your side naturally. To do this, try taking a deep breath. Bring your attention to how the chest expands and shoulders lift on the inhalation. Now bring your awareness to how the chest contracts and the shoulders and arms drop naturally at your sides.

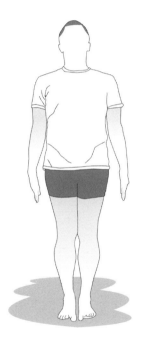

Therapeutic benefits:

Improves your posture.
Counteracts the degenerative effects of ageing on the spine, legs, and feet.

Uttanasana
(Standing Forward Bend Posture)

"Ut" means intense.

"Tan" means to stretch or extend.

In this posture I have noticed students trying to pull themselves with their upper body strength towards their legs, in the hope of bringing the torso to the thighs and stretching out the back of their legs. Often they end up with a sore back, tension around the shoulder and are no closer to releasing the hamstrings and enjoying the posture.

1. Bend your knees and fold your torso onto your thighs.

2. Keep your arms and elbows at your sides.

3. Bend the knees as much as you need to keep the fingertips in line with your toes.

4. Press down into the heels of the palms and forward through your fingers.

5. Lean the weight forward into the toes for a few breaths. Then lean the weight back into the heels.

6. Slowly start to straighten the legs. As the legs start to straighten bring your attention to the torso. As soon as the torso starts to leave the thighs, stop right there.

7. Now repeat step 2.

8. As the legs start to straighten, try to push the chin bones forward as you move the thighbones back. This action will help strengthen the entire leg, at the same time protecting your knee from hyperextension.

9. Remember to keep the hips parallel to the floor and extend the torso out of the pelvis.

Remember to use your breath. Inhale, lengthen the spine and exhale to move a little deeper into your posture.

Therapeutic benefits:
Relieves mental and physical exhaustion.
Improves digestion.
Stretches the backs of the legs and hips.
Stretches the lower spine.

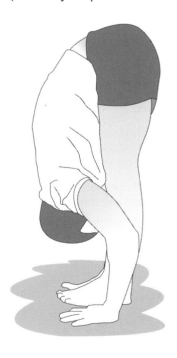

Vrksasana (Tree Posture)

"Vrksa" means tree.

Balancing postures develop our sense of balance and concentration. Keeping your eyes focused on a single spot, while moving with control and your breath, will help you find your balance on and off the mat. Remember this mantra: "slow, steady, control".

1. When balancing on one leg, make sure that you are standing on all four corners of your foot.
2. Bend your knee and then slowly straighten the leg. Press down into your heel and forward through your toes.
3. Keep a slight bend in the knee, to avoid hyperextension. Never lock out your knee, instead try to strengthen the muscles of the entire leg.
4. Move the shinbone forward as you move your thighbone back.
5. Transfer the weight onto the standing leg.
6. When placing the sole of the foot on the inner thigh, gently press the heel of the foot against the inner thigh as this will help with your balance.
7. Press the heels of your palms together, to help drop your shoulders away from the ears, and move the shoulder blades back into the body.

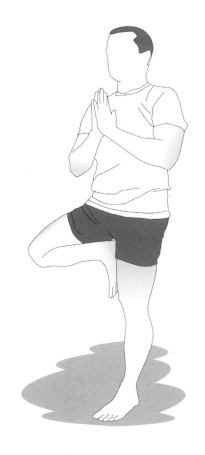

(...cont)

8. When lifting your arms, keep them in line with the centre of the chest. Follow the line upwards until the arms are straight.

9. Lift your chest to keep the spine straight.

10. Pick a spot on the floor, three feet in front of you, on which to focus your gaze. If this is too challenging at first, try balancing with the back of your body against wall. When you feel ready, move away from the wall.

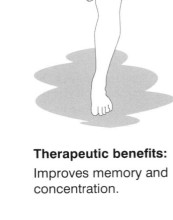

Therapeutic benefits:

Improves memory and concentration.

Utthita Trikonasana
(Extended Triangle Posture)

"Utthita" means extended.

"Tri" means three.

"Kona" refers to an angle.

In this posture the common problem that I have noticed is the placement of the feet. Too often I have seen students trembling, unstable and sometimes falling out of the posture. Because the stance is unsteady, students tend to collapse in the torso and take all the weight in their front leg and arm.

1. Try standing in Tadasana.
2. Take a step out to the right. Make sure that the outer edges of the feet are parallel, arms are shoulder level, stretched out and the fingers are together. Your wrists should be above and inline with your ankles.
3. Turn the right foot 90 degrees. Make sure the heel of the right foot is line with the inner arch of the left foot. If this stance is too challenging at first, try heel to heel.
4. Turn in the back foot 5 to 10 degrees.
5. As you extend to the right, slightly bend your knee, pressing the heel of the foot into the floor. Make sure you keep your knee inline with the centre of your foot. You can place the right hand on the shinbone or on the outside of the leg.

(...cont)

6.   If the hand is on the shinbone, press the shin against the hand in a forward motion. If the hand is on the floor, press down into the heel of the palm.

7.   Now slowly, straighten the right leg. This action will help ensure that the right hip moves towards the inner left heel.

8.   Press down on the outer edge of the back heel. This will assist balance and help distribute the work evenly on both legs.

9.   Start to slowly move the pelvis forward. Notice when the pelvis moves forward, your head moves back. This will allow you to open the chest upward. Keep in mind that if your top arm moves back, you will lose your alignment, so keep the top arm straight and inline with right arm. Remember to keep the fingers together and stretching up.

10. With the arm that is on the floor or shinbone, rotate the upper arm out. Notice when this happens, that there is more range of motion of the neck. Now look at your extended thumb.

11. Hold this posture for five breaths and then change sides.

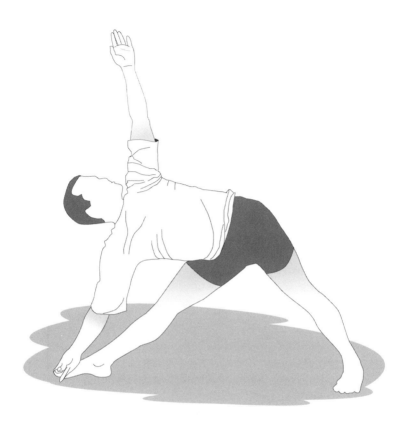

Therapeutic benefits:

Relieves gastritis, indigestion, acidity and flatulence.

Improves flexibility of the spine.

Alleviates backache.

Massages and tones the pelvic area.

Reduces discomfort during menstruation.

Adho Mukha Svanasana
(Downward-Facing Dog Posture)

"Adho" means downward.

"Mukha" means face.

"Svana" means dog.

This posture is the most recognised and relaxing of yoga postures. However, most people find this pose very challenging. Here are a few things to consider when in the pose.

1. Make sure your hands are shoulder distance apart and that the outer edges of your palms are parallel.

2. Your fingers should be spread wide, but not too wide, in order to prevent a strain on the wrists. A good rule to follow is that the middle finger should be facing the front of your mat with your thumb and index finger slightly turned in. You want to ensure that the whole hand is placed on the mat. Press down on the heels of your palms and forward, stretching through your fingers. Imagine that you are trying to push the floor away from you, keeping the arms straight.

3. Lifting your fingers and lowering them back to the floor will help to strengthen the forearm, thereby distributing the effort throughout the entire arm.

4. Most people will roll their shoulder blades together, restricting the space between the shoulder blades. Try to squeeze the outer edges of the armpits together and then release. Now roll your shoulder blades back into the body and towards your tailbone.

5. Now squeeze the forearms together, then release.

6. Lift your ribcage. One of the most common tendencies in this posture is to collapse into the ribcage, allowing the person to think that they are stretching out the spine. Try lifting the navel and ribcage and moving the lower ribs towards the thighs. This will allow the spine to straighten and lengthen.

7. Tuck in your tail. Another common misconception about this posture is that if you arch your lower back and lift your hips you will stretch the hamstrings. Try lifting the navel, lengthening the tailbone and pressing it in a forward motion. Now lift your sitting bones up. You will begin to stretch out the hamstrings and once again straighten and lengthen the spine.

8. Outer edges of the feet should be parallel. Lifting your toes and lowering them down creates an action in the legs that will help release your hamstrings, allowing you to bring the heels to the floor.

9. You can also bend your knees, lift your hips and slowly move towards straightening your legs, pressing the backs of the thighs to a wall, to help release the hamstrings.

10. To identify the actions of the legs, place a block between the thighs and squeeze the block.

(...cont)

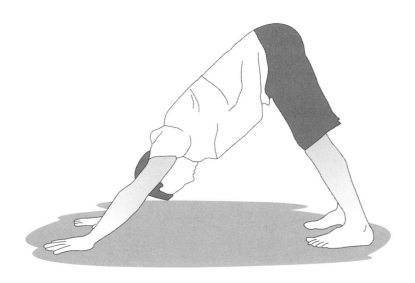

Therapeutic benefits:

Calms the brain and gently stimulates the nerves.

Slows down the heartbeat.

Strengthens the ankles and tones the legs.

Reduces stiffness in the shoulder blades and arthritis in the shoulder joints.

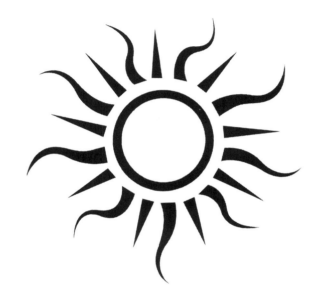

Seated Postures

All seated postures help to open the hips and provide mobility in the pelvis and increase the elasticity in the groin.

Dandasana (Staff Posture)

"Danda" means staff.

It is important to establish the correct actions in this posture, as it is the foundation of all seated postures. I have often found myself referring to the similar actions of this pose as I move into more deep-seated postures. You want to ensure that you are sitting on the sitting bones, the pelvis in a neutral position, the arms and spine straight. Here are few things to do:

1. Sit on the floor with the legs extended out in front of you.

2. Make sure you are sitting on your sit bones. To do that lean to one side and move the flesh out from each buttock.

3. Make sure the inner edges of the feet are touching. Now press the inner edges of the feet forward as the outer edges move back towards the hips.

4. Keep the heels pressed into the floor. This action will help you sit on your sitting bones.

5. Try to lift the shinbones off the floor. This action will engage the muscles in the legs allowing you to keep the backs of the legs on the floor. Now pull the legs back into the hip socket.

6. Try bringing the anklebones together. This will help you inwardly rotate the thighs.

7. Place the palms beside the hips and try pressing down into the palms and forward through the fingers. This action will help strengthen the entire arm. If the heels of the palms do not reach the floor, then move them forward just in front of the hips. Over time you can start to move the hands back.

8. Remember to roll the shoulder blades back into the body and towards your tailbone.

9. Slightly tuck your chin towards your chest to lengthen the back of the head.

10. Soften the gaze and jaw. Try placing the tip of the tongue on the roof of your mouth.

(...cont)

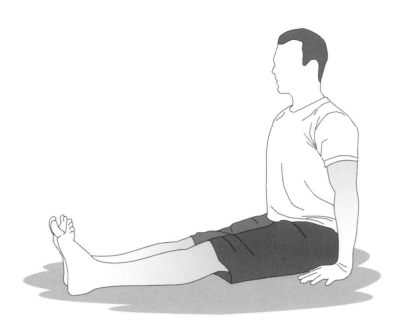

Therapeutic benefits:

Relieves breathlessness, choking, and throat congestion in asthmatics.

Strengthens the muscles of the chest.

Tones the abdominal organs and lifts sagging abdominal walls.

Reduces heartburn and flatulence.

Tones the spinal and leg muscles.

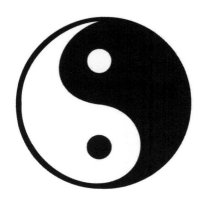

Forward Bends

Paschimottanasana (Intense West Stretch Posture)

"Paschim" means west.

"Uttana" means intense stretch.

This is one of the most relaxing and rejuvenating postures. I once held this posture for ten minutes and when I came out of it I felt as if I had slept for hours. Here are a few tips that will help you enjoy and deepen this posture:

1. The strength of this posture is your legs. Keep your legs straight and firm. Press the inner edges of the feet forward as the outer edges move back. Try to bring the anklebones together.

2. Press your heels into the floor. Press your sitting bones into the floor. This will allow your torso to extend out of your pelvis.

3. Keep the tops of the thighs spinning inward and at the same time pull the legs back into the hip socket. Make sure the bottoms of the thighs are pressed into the floor.

4. Start to lean forward from your hip joints not your waist.

5. Keep extending the torso out of the pelvis.

6. If you are unable to clasp the hands around the feet, then use a strap around the feet. Keep your legs firm and active. Hold on to the strap as you extend your torso out of your pelvis. Try to avoid pulling yourself forward with your arm strength. Instead, relax and roll your shoulders towards your tailbone. Use the strength and the actions of the legs and pelvis to fold forward.

7. If you can reach past your feet to clasp the hands, keep your arms straight.

8. Use the strength from your breath to move deeper into this posture. On your inhalation slightly lift your torso and on your exhalation release and extend into the posture.

9. When coming out of this posture, remember to inhale, lift your head and torso keeping your spine straight, and with your exhalation release your posture and return to Dandasana.

10. Hold this posture for five breaths.

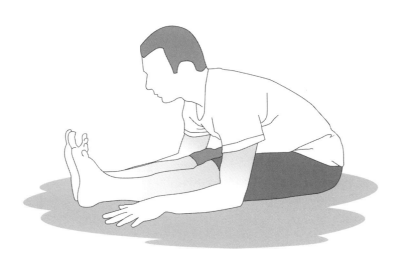

(...cont)

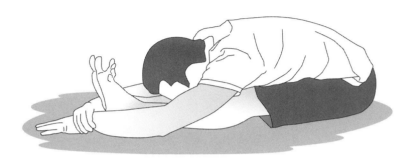

Therapeutic benefits:

Improves digestion.
Helps to stretch out the spine and hamstrings.
Stimulates the ovaries, uterus, and the entire reproductive system.
Tones the kidneys, bladder and pancreas.
Rests and massages the heart.

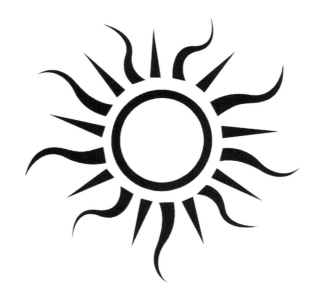

Janu Sirsasana (Head-to-Knee Posture)

"Janu" means knee.

"Sirsa" means head.

The next series of seated postures that we are going to look at are twists. Janu Sirasana is a great introduction as it is not only a forward bend but also a spinal twist.

One of the common things I have noticed happening to students in this posture is the misalignment of their hips, as well as the extended leg lifting off the mat and overstretching. Here are some things to think about in this posture.

1. Start in Dandasana.

2. Fold the right leg approximately 90 degrees, bringing the heel to the groin.

3. Top of the right foot, anklebone or knee, pressed into the floor, helping to ground the right sitting bone into the floor.

4. Place both hands on the floor approximately mid thigh of the extended leg. Then press down into the floor with both hands. As you do this, pull the extended leg back into the hip socket.

5. Make sure the extended leg does not roll out to the side or lift off the mat. Keep the thighbone pressed into the floor, press the inner edge of the foot of the extended leg forward as the outer edge moves back. Ground the left sitting bone into the floor.

6. Line up your navel with the inner line of the extended leg.

7. You can either place both hands on the shinbones or anklebones or reach around the foot of the extended leg to clasp the wrist.

8. With the strength of the legs, pelvis and your breath, start to extend the torso out of the pelvis.

9. As you lengthen forward, move the right side of the body towards the inner line of the left leg.

10. Square both shoulders. Make sure you do not pull yourself forward. Instead keep the spine straight, shoulders away from your ears, and keep extending forward.

11. Keep your elbows out to the side. If you are clasping your hands or wrist, gently pull the elbows to the sides to help broaden the chest allowing you to breathe freely.

12. Hold this posture for five breaths and then change sides.

(...cont)

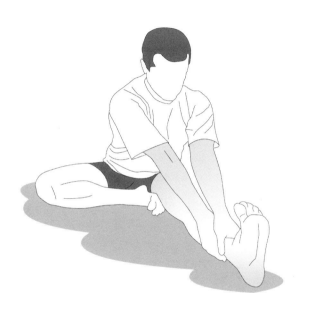

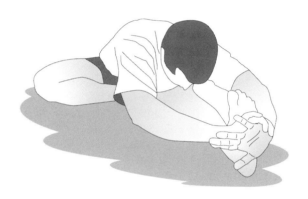

Therapeutic benefits:

Stretches the spine, shoulders and hamstrings.
Improves digestion.
Tones the abdominal organs.
Stabilises blood pressure.
Eases the effects of stress on the heart and mind.

Seated Twists

Twisting postures are energising, relaxing and a great way to release tension in your body. There are a few things to consider when you begin your twists. One is your foundation. In order to twist you need a counter weight to keep you grounded and anchored. It is important to try to keep your feet, legs, hips and sitting bones pressed into the floor, as they will be your foundation and act as a counter weight. With your foundation in place you can now begin to twist your spine in an upward motion.

Another thing to remember about twists is to keep your spine straight. Keeping your spine straight will help strengthen and develop the flexibility in your back. As your practice deepens you will increase the range of motion of your spine and eventually develop the control to isolate the action of twisting from the middle of your spine. Keeping the spine straight will also allow you to breathe more freely in a twisting posture. The breathing rule when twisting is, "inhale: lengthen your spine, exhale: twist."

Marichyasana (Spinal Twist Posture)

1. Sit in Dandasana.
2. Bend your right knee and bring your heel inline with your hip.
3. Turn in your right foot slightly. Remember to press down into the heel of your foot.
4. Place the fingertips of the right hand on the floor behind. Bring your bent knee to the centre line of your body. Straighten your back and lift your torso.
5. Lift your left arm in the air and turn your shoulders. Try to bring the outer edge of the armpit or the top of the arm against the right thigh.

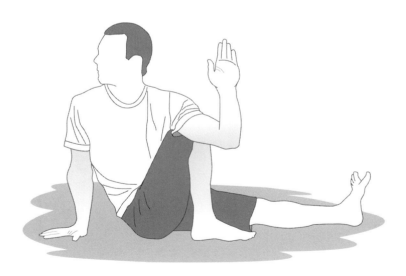

Now, depending on your flexibility, you can do either of two things.

1. You can straighten the left arm and press the back of the arm against the thigh. This will serve as a counter balance, help you rotate your torso and help the rounding of the back. As you rotate the torso around, start to walk the right hand around to the left buttocks. Turn your head and look over the right shoulder.

2. When you feel ready, you can bend your left elbow wrapping it around the right knee. Reach your right hand behind your back and grab your right fingers or wrist with your left hand.

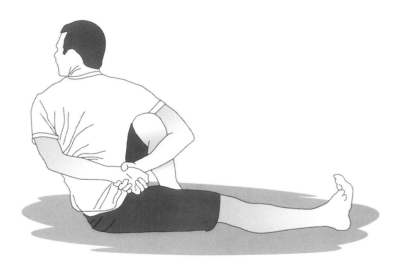

If you are unable to bend, try rotating the left shoulder forward and at the same time press the right thigh against the back of the arm. Notice how this action begins to deepen the twist.

If you are able to clasp your hands, then try pulling your elbows away from each other. This action will help stop the collapsing of the shoulders and rounding of the spine. Here is something to think about when it comes to wrapping the arm around the bent leg: you want to make sure that you clear your elbow around the leg so that you can bend it.

Remember to use your breath. Inhale, lengthen the spine and with your exhalation, twist deeper into your posture. Hold this posture for five breaths, and then change sides.

Therapeutic benefits:

Increases energy levels.

Tones and massages the abdominal organs.

Reduces fat around the waistline.

Alleviates backache.

Ardha Matsyendrasana
(Half Lord of the Fishes Posture)

"Ardha" means half.

"Matsya" means fish.

"Indra" means ruler.

This posture was originally named after a legendary yoga teacher.

This twist is one of my favourites, as it always leaves me feeling energised and relaxed. In this posture you can decide how deep you would like to go.

1. Sit in Dandasana.

2. Place your hands behind you, fingers pointing forwards. Now lean back on your hands. Cross the right leg over the left, placing the right foot on the floor, on the outer edge of the left knee. Now bend the left knee, sliding the left foot to the outer edge of the right hip.

3. Keeping your right hand on floor next to the buttocks, lift your left arm and torso. Rotate the torso to the right, placing the outer edge to the left armpit or the top of the arm against the right thigh. Keep the left elbow bent, with your fingers pointing towards the ceiling. Keep the fingers together. Now begin to twist. Look over the right shoulder. You can also vary the twist by keeping your gaze directly in front of you.

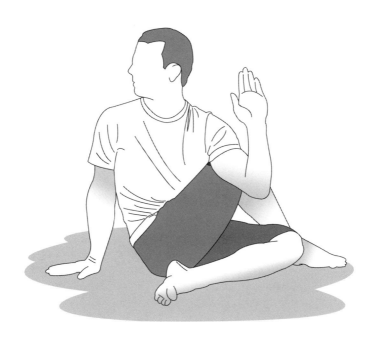

(...cont)

To deepen this posture here are a few variations that you can try:

1. Press down on the heel of the right palm.

2. Try bringing the left arm through the triangle of the right leg. Now reach around with the right arm and clasp either your hands or left wrist.

3. If you have clasped then gently pull the elbows away from each other to help deepen the twist.

4. Press the leg against the arm, dropping the outer edge of the hip on to the floor.

5. Press the heel of the right foot into the floor and at the same time press the outer edge of the right foot or anklebone into the floor.

6. Remember to move with your breath. Inhale, lengthen the spine, exhale, and twist.

By clasping your hands you can decide how deep you would like to twist.

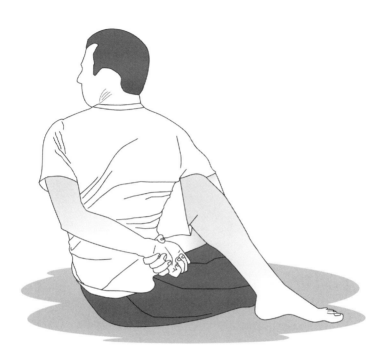

Therapeutic benefits:

Helps to stretch out the shoulders, hips and spine.

Helps relieve menstrual discomfort.

Provides energy and helps with fatigue.

Back Bends

Back bends are exhilarating, energising and one of the best ways to alleviate backaches. Back bends develop flexibility, and strengthen and increase the range of motion of the spine. In addition they open the chest, pelvic area and the entire front of the body. They are also one of the most challenging yoga postures. The reason for this is because we are constantly forward bending in our lives. For example, if something drops onto the floor, we don't bend backwards to pick it up, instead we bend forwards.

Sitting at a desk, hunched over, from Monday to Friday, nine to five, can lead to developing a rounded back as well as tightness in the upper back and chest. This daily routine is another reason why back bends are challenging. Having a flexible and strong spine is crucial to having a healthy spine and yoga practice. The following is a series of back bending postures that can help develop a healthy spine, strengthen the entire body and help end back pain.

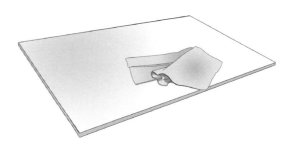

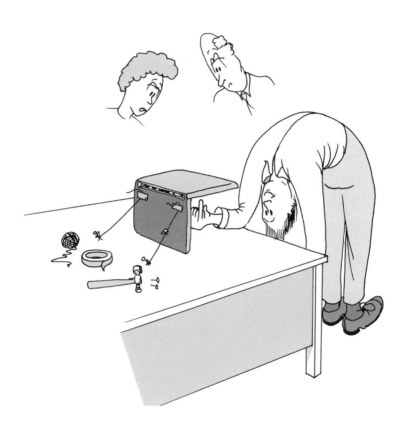

Bhujangasana (Cobra Posture)

"Bhujanga" means serpent or snake.

1. Lie on your mat face down. Place your hands by lower ribs. Your middle finger should be facing straight ahead. Your forearms should be vertical to your wrists.

2. Bring your awareness to your core and pelvic region. Lift the navel towards the spine and start to press your hips and outer edges of the pelvis into the floor. Remember to relax the buttocks by rotating the thighs inward.

3. Firm your legs by pressing the tops of the feet into the floor and lifting only your shinbones off the mat. This action will keep the legs active as well as relax the buttocks, freeing the pelvis to be pressed into the floor.

4. Now start to press down into the heels of the palms and forward through your fingers.

5. Keep the elbows at your sides. Roll the shoulders down away from your ears and shoulder blades back into your body towards your tailbone. This action will help lift the chest and increase the length of your neck.

6. Now start to lift your chest without using your arms, ensuring that you are using the strength of your spine to lift. Keep your elbows at your sides and continue to press down into the heels of your palms. Remember to lift your chest in an upward motion, instead of pushing it forward.

7. If this posture is too challenging at first, try placing your hands under your shoulders.

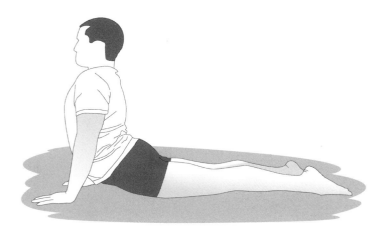

Therapeutic benefits:

Develops the strength of the spine.
Stretches and opens the chest, shoulder and the front of the body.
Relieves stress and fatigue and increases your energy levels.

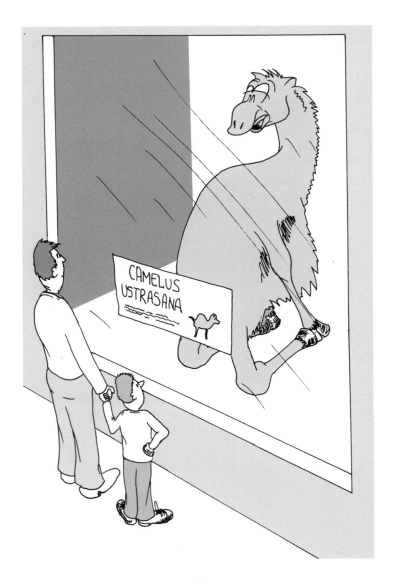

Ustrasana (Camel Posture)

"Ustra" means camel.

This posture is a great transitional posture between easier backbends and more challenging ones. Students of all levels can benefit from this posture because the full extension of the posture is easy for beginners to reach and it can be used as a preparatory pose for deeper back bends by advanced students.

1. Kneel on the floor with your hands on your buttocks, fingers pointing down. Your upper body should be upright and your spine straight.

2. For beginners, make sure your knees and feet are hip width apart. As your practice deepens you can bring the knees together. If the knees are hip width apart make sure your thighs and shinbones are parallel with one another.

3. Your feet should be pointing back. Lift and spread the toes.

4. Press the tops of the feet and shinbones into the mat. This will help identify the actions of the legs.

5. Start to squeeze your thighs together. This action will help you identify the inward rotation of the thighs.

(cont...)

6. Place your hands on your buttocks, with the heels of the palms at the top of the buttocks and your fingers facing down.

7. Lift the navel towards the spine and with your hands start to press the pelvis forward. Use your hands to help soften your buttocks.

8. Moving with your inhalation, start to lift your chest. Remember to roll your shoulders away from your ears and keep your shoulder blades pressed into your body.

9. Keep your chin pressed against your chest. This will help keep the length of your spine.

10. With control, begin to lower your hands towards your heels. If this is too far a reach then you can curl your toes under, placing the ball joints of the feet on the floor.

11. Place the heels of your palms on the heels of your feet with your fingers pointing towards your toes.

12. Roll the shoulders to the front and the shoulder blades towards the tailbone.

13. Continue to lift the navel towards the spine as you curl the pelvis up towards the ribcage.

14. Now let your head tilt back.

(cont…)

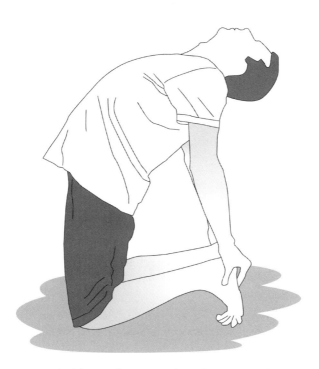

If you are not able to place your hands on your feet you can keep your hands on your buttocks, with the heels of the palms at the top of the buttocks and your fingers facing down. Now begin to bend back. As your practice deepens you can begin to lower your hands to your feet.

To come out of the posture, place your hands on your pelvis and start to push the pelvis forward. Keep the navel lifted and use the strength of your legs as you lead with your chest to lift out of the posture. Remember that your head will be the last thing to come up and out of the posture.

(...cont)

(cont...)

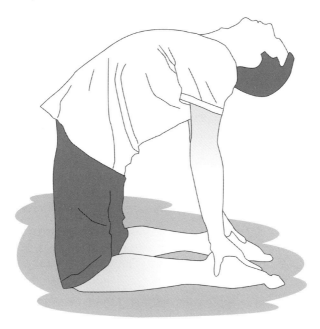

Therapeutic benefits:

Improves overall posture.

Stretches the entire front of the body.

Strengthens the muscles of the back as well as the spine.

Improves your breathing.

Relieves abdominal cramps.

Regulates menstrual flow.

Urdhva Dhanurasana
(Upward-Facing Bow Posture)

"Urdhva" means upward.

"Dhanur" means bow.

This posture, like the Downward-Facing Dog posture, is also one of the most recognisable yoga postures. This posture is energising, exhilarating and strengthens not only the back of the body, but the entire front of the body.

1. Start by lying on your back.

2. Bend your knees and bring your heels to your buttocks. Ensure that the legs are hip width apart and that the outer edges of the feet are parallel with one another.

3. Place the palms on the floor on either side of your head, with the fingers in line with your shoulders, and heels of the palms on the floor. Remember to keep your elbows parallel to each other.

4. Lift and spread your toes, lowering them back to floor. Now press your feet into the floor.

5. Press the heels of your palms into the floor. This will help with finding the arch in your upper back.

6. With your breath, start to lift your navel and pelvis, lifting onto the crown of your head.

7. As you press your feet into the floor, begin to lean the weight forward into your legs.

(...cont)

8. Start to straighten your arms. Remember to keep your forearms and elbows parallel to each other. Try squeezing your forearms and elbows together.

9. Remember in all back bends to keep the length throughout the entire spine. This will ensure that the bend will not be just in the lower spine but will be distributed evenly.

10. Take full deep breaths in your backbends. The common tendency in backbends is to either stop or speed up the breath. When moving into this posture use a deep inhalation and continue to breathe deeply and consciously.

11. To release this pose, start to bend your elbows, bringing the crown of your head to the floor. Now slowly lower your torso to the mat.

12. When you are finishing this posture, roll to the right and come to sit in Dandasana. Now fold forward into Pachismottanasana. This is a counter pose to your back bend.

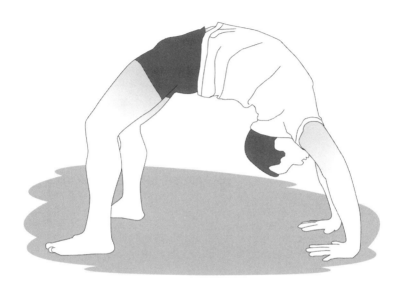

Therapeutic benefits:

Strengthens and develops flexibility of the spine.
Strengthens the arms, chest, abdominals and pelvic region, legs, and feet.
Is energising and helps with fatigue and stress.
Prevents the arteries of the heart from thickening and ensures healthy blood circulation throughout the body.
Helps to prevent excess menstrual flow and ease menstrual cramps.

Inversions

When you have completed your practice you will start on what is known as a Finishing Sequence. This is a sequence where your body will be inverted. By practising inverted postures, you will cool down your body, calm your brain and nervous system, and prepare yourself for final relaxation. In everyday life we are constantly in an upright position. This puts a lot of physical effort on us to provide blood to the upper parts of our body. By being inverted your brain, head, neck shoulders and chest are fuelled with blood.

The next two postures we will look at are shoulderstand and headstand.

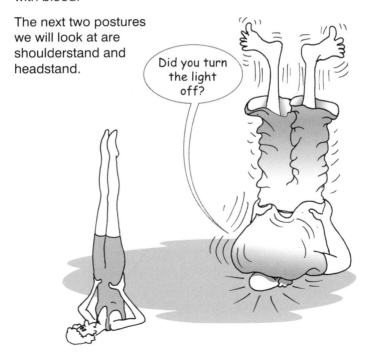

Niralamba Sarvangasana
(Shoulderstand Posture)

"Niralamba" means unsupported.

"Sarvanga" means all the limbs.

This posture is generally known as the Queen of all yoga postures. When practising this posture remember that you need to be on your shoulders and the back of your head and not your neck. Keep in mind this posture is called a shoulderstand. Any time you feel that you are on your neck, come out of the posture, readjust yourself and start again.

1. Lie on your mat, with your arms by your sides, palms pressed into the floor. Bring your anklebones together, keeping your legs firm.

2. Roll your shoulders back, bringing the shoulder blades back into the body. Start to press your shoulders into your mat.

3. Begin to press the palms into the floor. Lift your legs, hips and torso until your chest touches your chin. If this is too difficult at first, then you can bend your knees.

4. Now lean from side to side, once again rolling your shoulders back, and bringing the shoulder blades back into your body.

5. Bend your elbows and place your hands on the middle of your spine.

(...cont)

6. Now begin to lift the legs towards the ceiling. Remember to keep your body perpendicular to the floor.

7. Keep your elbows parallel to each other. Start to press the elbows and forearms into the floor.

8. Press your palms into your back to help straighten your body.

9. Try to bring your anklebones together and lift your navel towards your spine. This will keep your body feeling light.

10. Try not to let the legs move back and forth or to the sides. If this happens, then bend your knees and centre your waist with your chest and slowly lift your legs. If it continues to happen, then release the posture and start again.

11. Remember that your chest moves towards your chin, not chin towards the chest.

12. To release this posture, bend your knees towards your head. Place your palms on the floor and press down into the palms as you slowly roll out of the pose.

13. Lie and soften your body onto the floor.

Therapeutic benefits:

Improves the functioning of the thyroid and parathyroid glands.
Relieves insomnia and soothes the nerves.
Calms the brain and relieves mental sluggishness.
Improve blood circulation throughout the entire body.

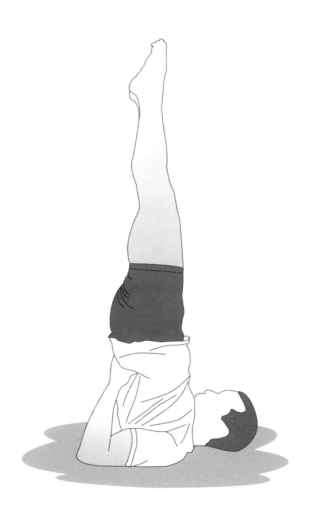

Salamba Sirsasana (Headstand Posture)

"Salamba" means supported.

"Sirsa" means head.

This posture also has a royal title. It is generally known as the King of all yoga postures. It is relaxing and very easy to do once you have mastered your balance. When first practising this posture, you might wish to start against the wall. Over time, when you feel comfortable, you can move away from the wall.

When starting this posture ensure that your foundation is secure. Placement of your hands, wrists and arms are important, as they will be your foundation.

1. Kneel on the floor. Place your elbows and forearms on the floor.

2. Make sure your elbows are shoulder width apart. Grab hold of the outer edges of your arms just above your elbows. This will help ensure that your elbows are directly under your shoulders. Keep your elbows in this position throughout the entire posture. If your elbows start to splay out, then stop and restart.

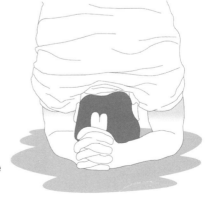

3. Clasp your hands interlocking your fingers; keep the inner edges of the thumbs pressing together.

4. Keep your wrists on the floor.

5. Roll your shoulders away from your ears and your shoulder blades back into your body and away from each other.

6. Start to press your forearms and elbows into the floor and forward. It should feel as if you are pushing the floor away from you.

7. Now place the crown of your head onto the floor, so that the back of your head touches your wrists.

8. Curl your toes under and lift knees off the floor.

9. Start to walk your feet in towards your torso, until you can't walk in further.

10. Still pressing down and forward into your forearms, elbows and wrists, lift your navel towards your spine and begin to lift your legs. Press the inner knees and anklebones together to help lift your legs.

11. If this is too challenging you can bend your knees towards your torso, lifting the feet off the floor. Now slowly straighten the legs. If this is still too challenging, try keeping one foot on the floor and lift one leg. Lower the leg down and change sides. Not only will this help you develop the strength to lift the legs but will also assist with balance, control, orientation and general comfort with being upside down.

12. You want to ensure that your hips are above the shoulders and that you never kick up into this posture.

(...cont)

13. If your knees are bent keep your heels close to the backs of your thighs as you begin to move your knees up and facing the ceiling. As you slowly straighten your legs, continue to gently press your inner knees together.

14. The legs should be perpendicular to the floor. One of the common tendencies in this posture is for the legs to twist towards the left or right. This usually happens when the position of the elbows has changed, in which case come down and reset your foundation and start again.

15. Once you have found your balance and you feel a general sense of lightness, hold this posture for at least 10 breaths. Once your practice deepens you can hold this posture anywhere from 5 to 25 minutes. The longer you hold this posture, the more your breath will start to deepen and slow down.

16. To come out of this posture you can keep the legs straight, bend at the waist and lower your legs. Keep your feet in a flexed position. This will help you slow or float down. Practising this exit out of the posture also helps with learning to lift or float your legs up.

17. When the feet are on the floor, place your knees on the floor, stretch your arms out, bring your hips to your heels and rest your forehead on the floor.

Therapeutic benefits:

Relieves the symptoms of colds, coughs and tonsillitis.

Improves the function of the pituitary and pineal glands.

Calms the brain and relieves mental sluggishness.

Develops concentration and focus.

Improves blood circulation throughout the entire body.

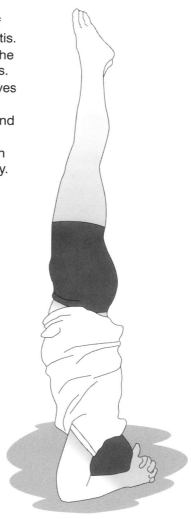

Savasana (Corpse Posture)

"Sava" means corpse.

This is the final posture of your practice and is often the most challenging posture. This is an active posture. Your goal is the ability to connect your mind and body while remaining calm and still. On many occasions I have seen people move and fidget around; and on several occasions students have fallen asleep and begun to snore in class. This is okay when starting out. This is a posture like any other, and when practised on a regular basis it will deepen over time. Be patient and consistent with this posture as it is also a time when the body starts to integrate all the work that you have done in your practice.

1. Begin by sitting in Dandasana.

2. Bend your knees and lean back on your forearms and elbows.

3. Lower your body to the floor. Straighten your arms, with your palms facing the ceiling.

4. Now begin to straighten your legs.

5. Begin an internal scan of your body.

6. Gently press the back of your head into the floor and then release. Remember to keep your head straight.

7. Roll you shoulders down away from your ears. Press your shoulder blades into the floor and then release.

8. Relax your core.

9. Let your feet fall out to the sides. Keep your body in a straight line.

10. Relax your jaw. Place the tip of your tongue on the roof of your mouth. Close your eyes and soften the muscles around them.

11. Relax your fingers and your toes.

12. Bring your awareness to your breath. Start to soften your breath. With your inhalation, feel your belly rise and with your exhalation it lowers.

13. Hold this posture for as long as you need. To come out of this posture begin to rotate your ankles and your wrists. Open your eyes and become familiar with your environment.

14. Bend your knees and roll to right, resting on your arm.

15. Place your left hand on the floor and push yourself up. Try to keep your head heavy and the last thing to come up.

16. Now sit for moment in a cross-legged position.

(cont...)

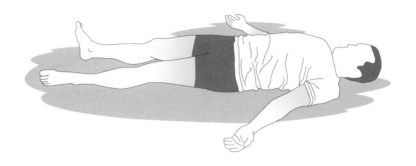

Therapeutic benefits:

Relaxes the body and eases breathing.
Soothes the nervous system and brings peace of mind.
Helps to alleviate nervous tension, migraines, insomnia
and chronic fatigue syndrome.

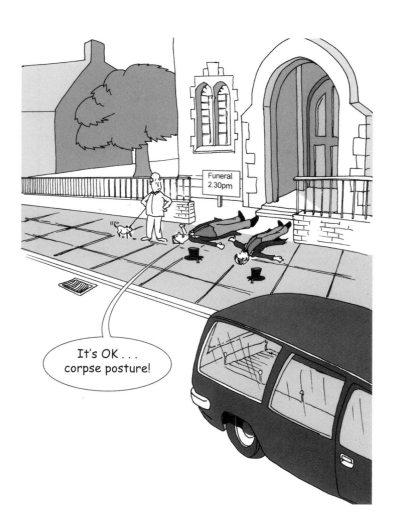

11. Pranayama - Breath Control

Pranayama is the practice of observing and ultimately controlling the breath, and is the fourth limb of Ashtanga, the eight limbs of yoga. Proper breathing controls the prana, or life energy, and goes hand in hand with our asana practice. Here are a couple of tips and techniques to introduce you to pranayama.

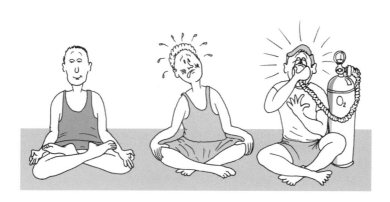

Find a comfortable seat

When you first try to sit for either pranayama or meditation, you will realise why we need to prepare with yoga asanas. It is hard to sit still for any length of time! At first, you will feel your legs cramp, or go numb, or you will feel an overwhelming urge to scratch, or before you know it, you will be slumped over with your chin almost on your chest. Oddly enough, it takes time to develop the ability to sit still.

Make it easier on yourself by getting comfortable when you sit. Sit on a mat or a blanket. Choose a position that you will be able to hold still. Full lotus is an ideal meditation pose, but few people can hold this position pain-free for more than a few minutes. It might be better to go with an easier position, like simply crossing the legs. Even then, you will find that any position can quickly become uncomfortable. If the discomfort is too much, and you are unable to relax, try sitting on a cushion or a block.

Let your back straighten, with your chin pulling slightly in towards your throat and your shoulders over your hips. Put your hand in your lap, or put the backs of your hands on your knees, with the tips of your index fingers and thumbs touching. Let the tip of the tongue rest lightly on the back of your top teeth.

(cont...)

The first few times that you sit, try sitting for just five minutes. You might be surprised by how challenging even five minutes of stillness can be. When you are able to sit absolutely still for five minutes, add one more minute onto your sitting time. Again, when you are comfortable with six minutes, add another minute, and continue in this way.

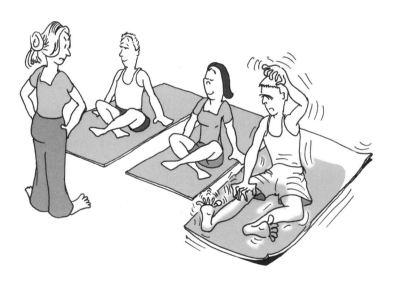

Kapalabhati

Kapalabhati is a basic pranayama that cleanses the body of mucus and builds an internal, purifying heat. "Kapala" means "skull", and "bhati" means "that which brings light", as this technique brings clarity to thought and a sparkle to the eyes. When doing this pranayama, make sure you end with some deep, slow breaths, and stop if you feel dizzy.

1. Sitting comfortably, take two normal breaths through your nose.

2. Inhale, and then sharply exhale through your nose, at the same time pulling in your abdomen.

3. Repeat up to twenty times, trying to keep a steady rhythm, and emphasizing each exhalation in the same way.

4. Inhale, then exhale completely, then inhale again and hold your breath for as long as is comfortable.

5. Slowly exhale, and take a few normal breaths.

6. Repeat two more times.

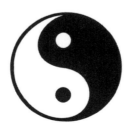

Belly Breathing

Our belly tends to hold tension when we are under stress. Tension in the belly can negatively affect our internal organs, our breathing, our digestion, and overall health. This pranayama relieves tension from the abdomen, and allows the diaphragm greater movement during inhalation and exhalation.

1. Sit comfortably, and take two normal breaths.

2. Bring your awareness to your belly. Letting it soften, take a long, easy inhalation and feel your stomach gently expand. Begin the inhalation at the base of the abdomen, and let the breath slowly fill the lower abdomen.

3. As you gently exhale, let your belly slowly contract from top to bottom, trying to keep it soft.

4. Try to keep your focus on your breath for as long as you can. When you tire, stop and take a couple of deep, normal breaths to finish.

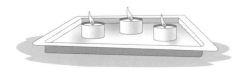

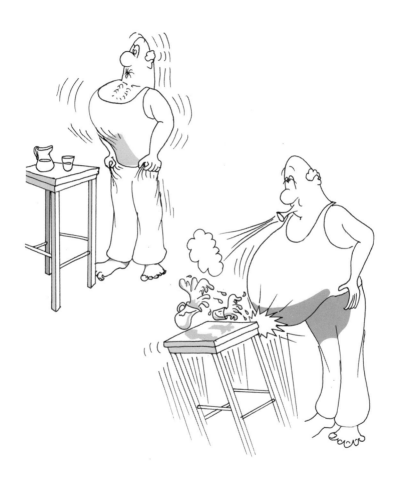

Ujjayi Breathing

Ujjayi breath is another pranayama that creates a purifying heat inside the body. To breathe Ujjayi you must partially close the throat, so that the breath makes a sound like a very gentle snore, or waves breaking on a distant beach. The sound should be easy, have a uniform pitch, and you want it to come from the throat, not the nose.

1. Sit comfortably and take two normal breaths.

2. Begin Ujjayi breathing, trying to make the inhalations and exhalations of equal duration and intensity. Inhalations should sound just like exhalations.

3. Try to keep your focus on your breath for as long as you can. When you tire, stop the Ujjayi breath and take a couple of deep, normal breaths to finish.

Health, Happiness and Peace of Mind

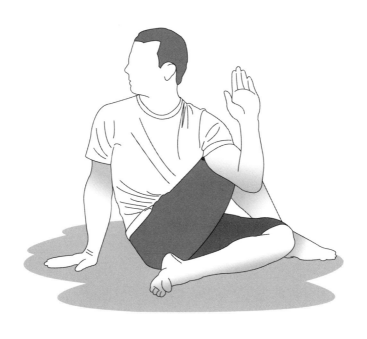

Half Lord of the Fishes

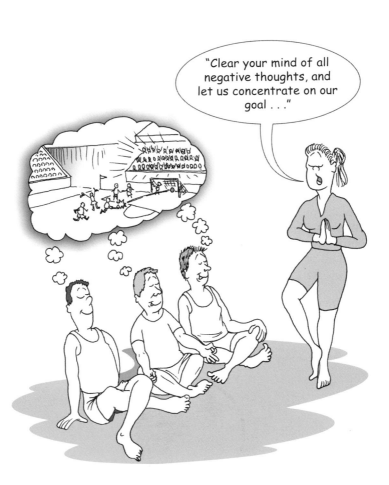

12. Meditation

Meditation occurs when moments of concentration seamlessly follow one another.
Meditation is the goal of our asana practice, and the seventh limb of Patanjali´s eight-limbed path. When we do yoga postures, we are creating and maintaining a healthy body, which provides a seat for a healthy mind. The practice of asana purifies our body and develops the inward gaze that is the basis of meditation. In a way, meditation spontaneously arises from concentration.

If you came to yoga for health reasons, you might not immediately be interested in meditating; perhaps it seems too abstract, or mumbo-jumbo. This definitely is not the case, as there are many different kinds of meditation, and some techniques are grounded and easily practised. Also, meditation has many physical benefits, as it can help us cope with stress and has been proved to benefit overall health and mental performance. Here are a couple of yogic meditation techniques, as well as tips on how to begin and deepen your meditation practice. See the tips on Pranayama for advice on sitting in meditation.

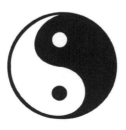

Concentration builds as we use it

Dharana is the practice of concentration, the sixth limb of Patanjali´s Ashtanga Yoga. When beginning to meditate it can be very difficult to stay focused. There are many different techniques to help train us to pay attention. To concentrate is to narrow our attention to a single point or category within our field of awareness. Practising concentration is how we build concentration. It is important to understand that the mind will wander, and that this is part of our training. Just the act of noticing that we are no longer focused is the act of building our focus. Try not to become discouraged, or distracted, by the difficulty of the task.

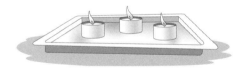

Tratak

Tratak is the practice of steady gazing, and is an excellent concentration exercise. To practise Tratak, you alternately gaze at an object or point without blinking, then close your eyes and visualise the object in your mind's eye. This technique gives us a solid co-ordinate for concentration, and trains us to focus our attention.

Tratak can be practised with any object as the focus, but I like using a candle. Here is how to practise:

1. Sit comfortably on a cushion or mat.

2. Place the candle three feet (90 cm) away from you, with the flame at eye level.

3. Calm your breath, and gaze at the flame without blinking. Try not to strain your eyes, just calmly watch the flame.

4. When your eyes get tired, close your eyes and visualise the flame with your inner-eye.

5. When the image of the flame becomes difficult to visualise, open your eyes and repeat.

Listen to your breath

Another great technique for concentration is focusing on the breath. When practising this technique, try counting your breath for the first minute. Count a slow four when you inhale, and do the same when you exhale. Any number will work, as long as the inhalation and exhalation are the same duration. Once the breath is steady, let yourself stop counting, and instead try to watch the breath as it moves in and out. Witness the sensations of the breath, without trying to control the breath. I find it easiest to focus by narrowing my awareness to the sensation of the breath as it passes the opening of the nostrils. When your mind wanders away from the breath, try not to chastise yourself or take any notice of what it is that distracted you, which will only create more distraction. Instead, gently bring your awareness back to rest on your breath.

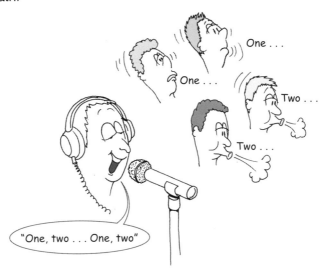

13. Kids' Yoga Tips

Yoga for kids is growing more popular. Kids really enjoy it, especially when they have a parent who practises, too. Kids receive the same benefits that adults do, like better body awareness, flexibility, co-ordination, and more self-control. Here are some tips for getting your kids to try yoga at home.

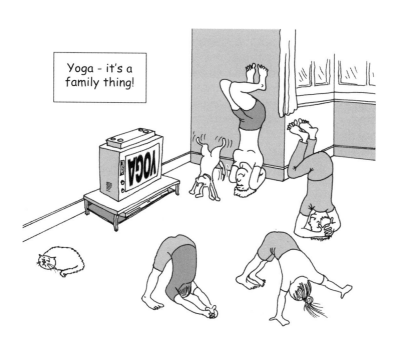

Make a special place to do yoga

Kids move around a lot, and they do not balance well for very long, particularly young children. Make sure that there is a lot of room for them to move around in. Kids do not necessarily need a mat, but they should have a designated space to do yoga in. It helps if the space provides some support for balancing poses, like a wall or soft chair.

Start with breathing

Do a breathing exercise at the beginning of the child's yoga session to help them connect with their breath. Belly Breathing is a great breathing exercise. Either sitting or lying down, the child places their hands on their belly, and inhales the belly out, exhale belly in. Reversing the movements of the belly also works, pulling the belly in on the inhalation, and pushing the belly out on the exhalation.

Focus less on enlightenment, more on having fun

Let children find their own benefits when they practise yoga. Telling them how they should feel limits their experience. Do not bog down children by trying to keep yoga serious. Instead, stimulate their interest by making the poses fun. Many poses are named after animals, so be playful, and bark in Downward-Facing Dog, hiss in Cobra, and roar in Lion Posture. Encourage input from the children; get them to teach you yoga poses too, as this gets them more involved.

Move through the poses quickly

Most children have short attention spans, and it can be difficult for them to hold still. Instead of holding poses for any length of time, try flowing through many different poses, and limit the class to 15 or 20 minutes. Never force a child's body into a pose; let them try to find the pose in their own way. Teach the kids a simple Sun Salutation that you can come back to whenever they get restless.

Guided relaxation

Kids love relaxation pose. End each yoga session by dimming the lights and encouraging the children to get comfortable. Do not worry about what position they lie in, as long as they are relaxed. Begin to deepen their relaxation with belly breathing or calming music.

Take the children to even deeper relaxation through visualisation. Get the children to envision doing a favourite activity, or take them on an imaginary walk through the woods, spotting wildlife and plants. At the end of the relaxation, encourage the children to share their experiences.

14. Prenatal Yoga Tips

Prenatal yoga is extremely popular, and so it should be. Yoga is the perfect way to stay in shape during pregnancy, as it keeps expectant mothers limber and fit, improves balance and circulation, and all without any negative impact on the joints. Yoga also helps pregnant women learn to relax and breathe deeply, preparing them for the physical demands of labour, birth, and motherhood.

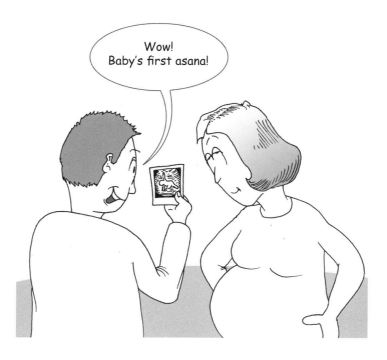

Check with your doctor or midwife before starting your yoga programme

If you already have a yoga practice, you can probably continue to practise with modifications while you are pregnant, provided your pregnancy is not considered high risk. Check with your doctor or midwife to make sure that yoga will still be safe for you.

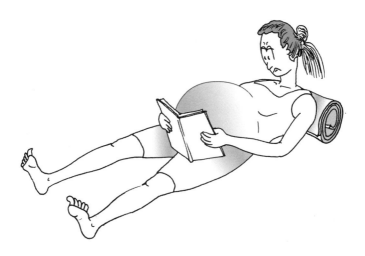

Get the right teacher

If possible, find a teacher specifically trained in prenatal yoga, or make sure your own teacher knows that you are pregnant. Some types of yoga should not be practised in the first trimester. If you ever feel pain or discomfort during class, ask your instructor to recommend an alternative position.

Modify your practice

You need to change your practice when you are pregnant. If you have an existing practice, accept that you will have to change this to accommodate your developing pregnancy. Modify as you need to, and drink water before, during and after your practice to stay hydrated. Be careful of overdoing a stretch, as your joints will get looser later in your pregnancy.

Use props as you get bigger. You can use the wall or a chair for balancing poses, and blocks and straps in any of the other poses.

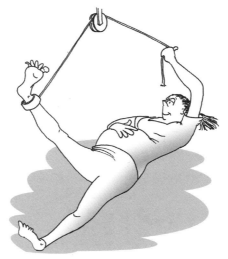

Squat

Squatting is a great way to prepare your hips for giving birth. Squat every day, using props to support yourself when you get bigger. When you get too big to squat, try sitting poses.

Poses to avoid

There are some asanas that you should not do when
you are pregnant. Sometimes lying on your back can
be a problem after the first trimester. If you have never
done inversions like shoulderstand and headstand, you
should not attempt them when pregnant. If you have an
established practice, then inversions are fine up until the
third trimester. Avoid poses like deep forward and back
bends as it is much easier to tear muscles when pregnant,
due to changes in the hormones. Deep twists should also
be avoided, and any pose that puts pressure on your
stomach, from the beginning of your pregnancy onwards.

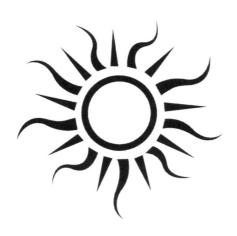

15. Postnatal Yoga Tips

If you are a new mother, then you are probably getting plenty of activity: lifting, bending and carrying. Still, you may want to be a little more focused about where you are getting your exercise, or you may want to restart a pre-existing yoga practice. Yoga is the perfect tool to help you deal with the challenges and stresses of being a new mother.

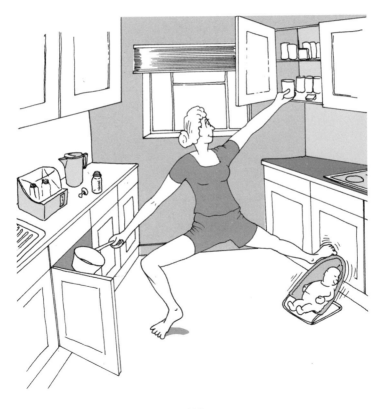

Give yourself time

If you were already practising yoga before you had a baby, then try to resume your practice as soon as you have some time, but do not expect to start practising again for about a month. And when you do begin to practise, make sure you go very slowly and avoid strain. This is your chance to take your time, and can be an opportunity to reapproach your practice.

Focus on restorative yoga

After giving birth, it is best to do a restorative practice for a little while. Use props like a blanket and pillows to support your poses, and focus on releasing tension without creating strain. The benefits of this practice will extend beyond the renewed energy and calm you will feel, as your child will also sense when you are tired and stressed, or calm and centred.

Join a class

Many studios offer "Mother and Baby" yoga classes. These classes are not only an opportunity to get into shape and connect with your baby, but also a chance to meet other new mothers with similar interests

Start with ten minutes

It can be very difficult to resume a practice, not to mention now having to find the time between feeding and naps. A good trick is to start off in very small increments, and work from there. If you put too much pressure on yourself, yoga will seem like one more task, and not the potential oasis in your day that it can be. Give yourself just ten minutes for the first few weeks that you restart your practice, and then slowly increase the time that you spend on the mat.

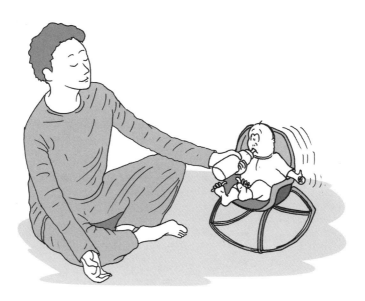

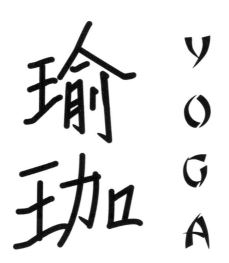

瑜珈 YOGA

16. Yoga Etiquette

Turn off the cell phone

I know that you *meant* to turn off your cell phone, but what with being in a rush, trying to find a spot for your mat, and having to get changed, you forgot. And now, just as we are entering into deep relaxation, your phone has started ringing. And that is okay. It is not ideal, but it is okay.

It is *not* okay to let the phone ring because you are too embarrassed to get up and turn it off. It is not okay to make the class listen to the phone ring, and ring, and ring.

Your best course of action: get to your phone as quickly as possible. *Do not answer it*. ("Hello? No, I'm at yoga… Yoga!") Just turn it off, apologise, and return to your mat. All is passing.

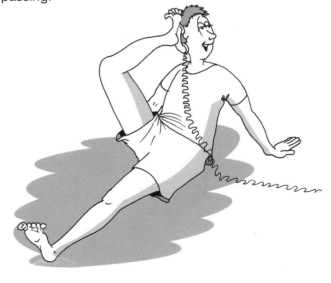

Do not leave during Savasana

Unless you are trained as a ninja, you are going to disturb the entire class when you leave in the middle Savasana. If you have to go early, plan on leaving before the class lies down for the final relaxation posture. Give yourself five minutes before you leave to lie back and relax, and then, when the class is preparing to take Savasana, quietly slip out.

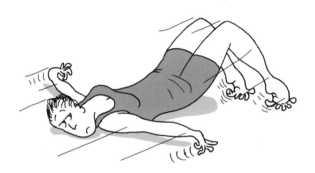

Know when to speak up

Good teachers always appreciate feedback from students. They will listen carefully when a student tells them what they liked, or did not like, about a class. Generally, teachers like the feedback after but not during the class. It can be very distracting for other students when someone repeatedly makes comments during class, either to the teacher or other students. The exception to this is when a student is receiving an adjustment, or push, in a posture from the teacher; it is very important to let the teacher know if an adjustment is causing pain.

Avoid wearing perfume or 'No common scents!'

Before your class, rinse off any perfume that you might be wearing. While you may have not have put on much perfume, as you warm up, any scent that you have on is going to diffuse throughout the room. That sweet smell will become a noxious cloud, choking your teacher and fellow students. Also, some people have sensitivities to certain chemicals, and might develop a more severe reaction. Remember, some skin lotions and shampoos also contain perfumes — start buying unscented products.

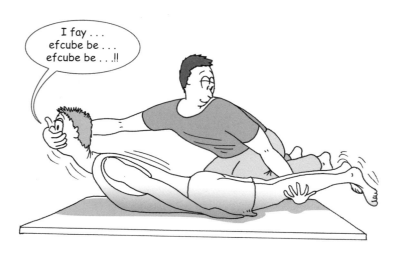

17. Yoga Jokes and Sayings

Q: How many Iyengar yogis does it take to change a light bulb?

A: Just one, but he is going to need a chair, two blocks, and a strap.

*

Change is inevitable, except from vending machines.

*

Three yogis in a cave…

…sit meditating, when there is a loud "boom" outside the cave. Five years later, one of the yogis says "That sounded like a battle". Another five years pass, and a different yogi says "I think it was thunder". Ten more years pass and the third yogi says "If you guys do not stop bickering, I am leaving!".

*

Q: Why couldn't the yogi vacuum his carpet?

A: He had lost his attachments.

*

Blessed are the flexible, for they shall not be bent out of shape.

*

Q: What did the sign in the window of the yoga studio say?

A: Enquire within!

*

Time is the best teacher, although it kills the students.

Glossary of Yoga Terms

Ahimsa - non-harming, the first and most important moral discipline, or yama.

Asteya - non-stealing, which is one of the ethical guidelines, or yamas, in Patanjali's eight-limbed yoga.

Aparigraha - noncovetousness, which is one of the ethical guidelines, or yamas, in Patanjali's eight-limbed yoga.

Asana - a physical posture, literally means "seat"; the third limb of Patanjali's eightfold path.

Ashtanga Yoga - the eight-limbed yoga of Patanjali, consisting of ethical restraints (yama), spiritual discipline (niyama), posture (asana), breath control (pranayama), sensory withdrawal (pratyahara), concentration (dharana), meditation (dhyana), and enlightenment or union (samadhi).

Ayurveda - a traditional science of Indian medicine.

Brahmacharya - the discipline of sexual continence, which is one of the ethical guidelines, or yamas, in Patanjali's eight-limbed yoga.

Chakra - a wheel; one of the psycho-energetic centres of the subtle body.

Dharana - concentration, the sixth limb of Patanjali's eight-limbed yoga.

Dhyana - meditation, the seventh limb of Patanjali's eight-limbed yoga.

Dharma - law or virtue.

Guru - a spiritual teacher.

Hatha Yoga - a path of yoga that emphasises asana and pranayama.

Ishvara pranidhana - surrender to God / The Universe. One of the spiritual disciplines, or niyama, in Patanjali's eight-limbed yoga.

Karma - activity of any kind that accumulates when performed in a self-centred way.

Karma Yoga - the spiritual path of self-transcending actions.

Nadi - one of 72,000 or more channels through which life force, or prana, circulates.

Namaste - a greeting, which basically means "I bow to you."

Niyama - spiritual discipline, or self restraint. The second limb of Patanjali's eight-limbed path, which consists of cleanliness (saucha), contentment (samtosa), discipline in practice (tapas), study (svadhyaya), and surrender to God / The Universe (ishvara-pranidhana).

Om - a mystic word, or mantra, regarded as the root of all sounds and letters, and the origin of all language and thought.

Prana - the life force that sustains the body.

Pranayama - breath control, the fourth limb of Patanjali's eight-limbed path.

Pratyahara - withdrawal of the senses, the fifth limb of Patanjali's eight-limbed path.

Sadhana - spiritual discipline.

Samadhi - the state of union, the eighth and final limb of Patanjali's eight-limbed path.

Samsara - the world of change.

Samtosa - contentment, one of the practices of spiritual discipline, or niyama, in Patanjali's eight-limbed yoga.

Satya - the practice of truthfulness, which is one of the ethical guidelines, or yama, in Patanjali's eight-limbed yoga.

Saucha - cleanliness, one of the practices of spiritual discipline, or niyama, in Patanjali's eight-limbed yoga.

Shanti - peace.

Siva - the Destroyer, the god of yoga.

Sthira bhaga - means "divine stability" and is often used as a greeting.

Svadhyaya - study, one of the practices of spiritual discipline, or niyama, in Patanjali's eight-limbed yoga.

Tapas - heat, discipline in practice, one of the practices of spiritual discipline, or niyama, in Patanjali's eight-limbed yoga.

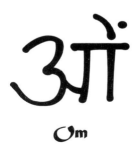

Om

Index

Index

Index

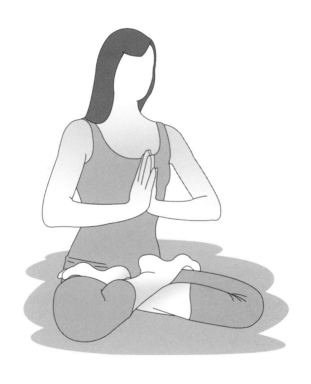

Lotus

Space for your thoughts . . .

Space for your thoughts . . .

Space for your thoughts . . .